The Advanced Dom's Guide To Submissive Training

42 Must-Know Tips To Make You The Billionaire DOM That No Sub Can Resist. A Must Read For Any Dom/Master In A BDSM Relationship

Elizabeth Cramer

Copyright© 2016 by Elizabeth Cramer

The Advanced Dom's Guide To Submissive Training

Copyright© 2016 Elizabeth Cramer
All Rights Reserved.

Warning: The unauthorized reproduction or distribution of this copyrighted work is illegal. No part of this book may be scanned, uploaded or distributed via internet or other means, electronic or print without the author's permission. Criminal copyright infringement without monetary gain is investigated by the FBI and is punishable by up to 5 years in federal prison and a fine of $250,000. (http://www.fbi.gov/ipr/). Please purchase only authorized electronic or print editions and do not participate in or encourage the electronic piracy of copyrighted material.

Publisher: Living Plus Healthy Publishing

ISBN-13: 978-1530966592

ISBN-10: 1530966590

Disclaimer

The Publisher has strived to be as accurate and complete as possible in the creation of this book. While all attempts have been made to verify information provided in this publication, the Publisher assumes no responsibility for errors, omissions, or contrary interpretation of the subject matter herein. Any perceived slights of specific persons, peoples, or organizations are unintentional.

This book is not intended for use as a source of legal, business, accounting or financial advice. All readers are advised to seek services of competent professionals in the legal, business, accounting, and finance fields.

The information in this book is not intended or implied to be a substitute for professional medical advice, diagnosis or treatment. All content contained in this book is for general information purposes only. Always consult your healthcare provider before carrying on any health program.

Table of Contents

Introduction 3

Chapter 1: The Billionaire Mindset - A Lesson in Dom Seduction 5

    How to Look Like a Billionaire with Just Five Dollars in Your Pocket 10

Chapter 2: How to Turn an Innocent into Your Sexual Slave 13

    The Qualities of a Sexy Teacher 15

    Become a More Charismatic Seducer 17

    And Here's How You Take Someone to Bed 19

Chapter 3: A Guide to Becoming More Confident as a Dom 21

Chapter 4: How to Pass a Sub's Tests 29

Chapter 5: Three Hour Foreplay and Aftercare 37

    Preparing the Sub as Part of Foreplay 43

Positions Commonly Used 46

Classwork and Homework........................ 51

The More the Merrier 57

Chapter 6: How Many Ways Are There to Enjoy Intimacy?... 61

Chapter 7: Live Like a Sub to Discipline Like a Dom.. 79

The Six Subs You Meet............................... 82

Common Mistakes Made by Dums (Not Doms!).. 85

Putting on the Mind of Your Partner 88

How to Draw Out a Shy Sub 92

Chapter 8: How to Put Your Partner in a Sexual Trance... 95

Chapter 9: How to Use BDSM Practices to Heal Someone's Pain................................ 101

Helping the Sub with Long-Term Beneficial Discipline 104

Conclusion 109

Other Books by Elizabeth Cramer 111

Introduction

We're glad you've joined us for another book in our BDSM series, how to become a Dom and master the lifestyle. This education is going to help you become a better Dom, a better leader and a better trainer for these subs who are looking for strong guidance in their lives.

In this book, we're going to focus on becoming a "billionaire" type of Alpha Dom so that you can become more attractive to the subs you offer your services to. It's very timely, of course, with all these BDSM Billionaire erotica books being released. However, you are soon going to find out that money actually has nothing to do with the attraction the Dom builds with the sub. It's all in personality, in posturing and in a certain way of thinking.

We're going to train you, Dom to Dom, how to activate that attraction and more importantly how to come across as a worldly-wise educator to a sub that needs someone strong, smart and creative in her life.

For the sake of simplicity, as with the other books in this series, all Doms are referred to as He and all subs are referred to as She. However, sexes are interchangeable. All that matters is that you are determined to become an advanced level Dom and willing to do the work that goes along with the title and prestige.

So let's get started in training you to become:

- Alpha
- Dominant
- Valuable
- Educated
- Confident

And the famous "billionaire" charm that will make you irresistible!

Let's begin with Chapter 1.

Chapter 1: The Billionaire Mindset - A Lesson in Dom Seduction

It's no coincidence that popular BDSM literature seems to feature "alpha billionaires," that is, men who are dominant, rich and not so coincidentally desired by women. While it's true this is a book/movie cliché it is worth exploring for psychological insight.

Billionaires, unlike most "average men", have what you call instant value. If a very attractive woman has "commodity" in her beauty, then a billionaire's commodity would be his lifestyle. His ability to go anywhere in the world, spend mad money and take off work whenever he'd rather be skiing or wave-riding. This is elementary when it comes to the lure of seduction.

The seducer has "commodity" and so it's very easy for the person who has something of value to seduce a person who is in need. This applies to BDSM Dom discipline as well.

Tip #1: The Dom should always demonstrate value.

Of course, it's safe to assume you're not Christian Grey or even Donald Trump, when it comes to making that kind of money. Most people don't, and the idea that it's easy to become rich and famous is obviously far-fetched. However, a lack of financial resources doesn't mean you are incapable of demonstrating your commodity, or your value.

You can still demonstrate the attractive qualities billionaire archetypes possess. For instance, your average billionaire is:

- Super-confident, almost to the point of arrogance

- Not afraid of losing anything or anyone, because getting more is always easy

- Has a certain "impress me" attitude that most men don't have

- Has entitlement to do or say almost anything

And of course, a billionaire gets away with being arrogant and ballsy, because he's got that hot commodity. As a non-billionaire, obviously you won't have the same level of leverage or star-power to get away with as much. Still, women and really all "subs" regardless of gender, will respect a Dom who acts like a billionaire.

Tip #2: A Dom feels "entitled" to do or say things that ordinary men would not.

This entitlement MUST be part of your MO as a Dom, because a sub is counting on you to be aggressive, motivated and to make very specific requests of her, so that she doesn't have to over-think things. Submission is all about letting go of power and getting in touch with unconscious, deeply rooted feelings.

Therefore, your priority in learning to be a powerful Dom who influences your subs with ease, will require that you demonstrate your value and your best "Features," while also showing your Alpha Dom personality.

The first part is relatively easy. You may not be rich but you accentuate your favorable trails:

1. Good looks

2. Intelligence

3. Charisma or charm

4. Sexy voice

5. Muscular body

6. Creativity

7. Vivid imagination

8. Talents or abilities

9. Good at reading people and giving them what they want

10. An experienced "Dom" in the lifestyle

All of these are positive traits that you can highlight when conversing with your sub for the first time. Naturally, you don't want to "tell" your sub that you're such a great Dom. That's selling and it creates resistance. Rather, you want to show – you want to demonstrate this with your body language, your conversation and your mental prowess.

Your entitlement is really all about being an Alpha and not letting the sub dominate the conversation. While it is true that subs ultimately have all the control in a BDSM relationship, you, the Dom, are the one who should dominate the conversation and the relationship flow.

Tip #3: The Dom comes up with ideas. The Dom thinks of something to say. The Dom draws out the sub in conversation. The Dom is assertive in leading the conversation.

In other words, be *entitled*. Be confident in yourself and unleash your TRUE SELF, not the polite, politically correct version that you think people want. Work on showcasing your talents and gifts in regular conversation and on leading people in conversation. Not knowing what to say or do, is really the sub's prerogative. After negotiation, your creativity is taxed.

Doms are never actually required to be "nice." In negotiation, yes, you owe it to your sub to be honest, to be polite and to be professional – and not come across as a psychopath. However, once you become a Dom and the scene begins, your priority is discipline, not being nice. Not showing her a good time. Not pleasing her or giving her what she "wants."

The priority is teaching her something, disciplining her according to what she NEEDS, according to what she needs to FEEL.

How to Look Like a Billionaire with Just Five Dollars in Your Pocket

It's no coincidence that many famous millionaires have similar personality traits. In almost every profile, you read you will see that these individuals were:

- Risk-takers

- Ambitious

- Always coming up with ideas

- Persistent

- Focused on what the market wanted

So in presenting your Dom personality to your sub, even during the negotiation phase, ask yourself these questions.

- "Am I coming across as too safe? Too nice? Or am I communicating power and confidence in my own abilities?"

- "Do I seem like a person who might become great some day? Do I have big goals and big dreams? Or do I just seem like a person wanting sex?"

- "Am I an active thinker, always coming up with ideas?"

- "Am I tough and tenacious or do I give up too easily?"

- "Am I just trying to satisfy myself or am I thinking of what my Subs want?"

Just imagine if you were a billionaire. Visualize winning the lottery or writing a best-selling book. Now ask yourself, how has your personality changed now that you're successful and well known? What flaws did you eliminate in yourself now that you don't "need" anybody's approval? Has your tolerance for certain negative behaviors in others decreased? Do you have higher standards?

Tip #4: The Dom always has a high set of standards, because the sub must be trained to meet them.

The sub cannot reach your lofty standards, not at first. You are not lucky to have the sub.

The sub desires you because of your commodity; you are an alpha Dom; a man (or woman) who is mentally rich and entitled.

Your sub may be beautiful, and you may even tell her that if you choose, but you must never put the sub on a pedestal. Spoiled little princesses never "learn". They must be taught not to take things for granted.

The Dom has very high standards and this is usually what creates attraction in subs, since they desire discipline, training and protection or some type of sustenance—whether that's physical or mental.

In the next chapter, we're going to explore just how that Billionaire Alpha Male always manages to seduce the young and naïve beauty. And it's never about money.

Chapter 2: How to Turn an Innocent into Your Sexual Slave

In most BDSM related literature, the Dom doesn't actually use any of his money to win the affection of the young lover. Instead, it's his personality, his resonating mind that impresses her. His money may be the attention-grabber, but his alpha persona is what creates the attraction.

"Alphas" in the wild mean leaders of the "pack" or in a tribe of animals. Some alphas win the power by being aggressive, but usually it's the alpha that has the most superior abilities that assumes a leadership role. The reason being, because following him is beneficial to the entire tribe or pack. He's smart, he's strong, and he knows how to protect the entire community. And of course, the females all want the alpha male because his genetics are superior and she can anticipate a higher quality of offspring.

That's more valuable than just aggression. Of course, most alphas who have greater abilities are naturally aggressive.

There you have the billionaire formula. You are attractive to "subs" (the submissive partners) because you have a superior mind. You are the teacher, the trainer and the mentor. THAT is what Subs, especially young and beautiful ones, find irresistible.

Tip #5: Always strive to be the teacher, not the FOLLOWER.

If you want to be sub, then that's when you would try to impress the Alpha with your "commodity"; usually your innocence, your virginity, your sex appeal, etc. However, for a Dom, you MUST show yourself to be a strong-minded teacher.

Teachers are naturally confident, maybe even entitled. They are head of the class and their students are there to learn for their own benefit. This instantly gives the teacher power and entitlement to control the classroom and to control the students. The teacher is not only assertive when it comes to demanding obedience—he also has a structured curriculum to teach. Which brings us to…

Tip #6: Always have a plan of action ready to go. If you don't, you will lose confidence.

Curious? Try teaching a class a new subject if you have no idea what the subject is. It's painful, it's embarrassing and it's just a disaster, right? Same way with trying to be a Dom without having a specific plan of action.

This involves finding out what the sub wants and then creating "scenes" that give the sub the training she needs. This creates the cohesive structure to your discipline that you need to stay focused.

The Qualities of a Sexy Teacher

Tip #7: If you're unsure of how to play the "teacher," then re-familiarize yourself with essential Alpha Teacher qualities that students find attractive.

They are fairly basic and most students will "fall" for these qualities time and time again, because they are mentally and emotionally attractive.

1. Engaging way of speaking and creative methods of teaching

2. Clear objectives demonstrated at the outset (what the Sub needs to learn and why)

3. Strong disciplinary mind (not necessarily abuse, just firm discipline)

4. Teaches a student self-improvement in training (in stark contrast to just repetitive abuse)

5. Always has high expectations in the student, pushes a little hard so the student will achieve beyond their own expectations

6. Knowledge of the subject matter (which is why experience and training in BDSM equipment and toys is important at this stage)

7. And once again…trust!

The first of these is the most important, since obviously if you lack charisma you will never be a good "seducer" or a good teacher, and ultimately never a Dom. A Dom has to be charismatic.

Tip #8: Take steps to improve your own charisma.

No question, a charismatic Dom is always going to be a popular guy – versus a guy who just craves sex and has little personality.

What are the keys to becoming more charismatic? It doesn't just apply in BDSM theory but in all of life.

First, consider the mechanical aspects of charisma.

Become a More Charismatic Seducer

1. Work on manipulating your voice to be more exciting:

    - Higher and lower pitches for emotional statements

    - A faster way of speaking for intense statements

    - A slower way of speaking for emotional peaks

    - Greater volume to emphasize statements of power and meaning.

2. Be self-confident.

   - Learn to like yourself and stop doubting or thinking that the other person finds you unattractive. Believe that they do.

   - Be enthusiastic, positive and happy.

   - Don't mix your Dom fun with your own personal issues in life. You're the DOM not the SUB. It's not about YOU.

   - Maintain strong eye contact. Never cower. You don't have to stare, but you're never afraid to make a connection.

3. Learn a little bit more about the world. Learn something new and interesting to say.

4. Maintain open body gestures; open arms and comfortable legs. Avoid crossing your legs and arms or anything else defensive.

5. Smile naturally but don't always smile and don't fake-smile. Keep it honest. You may also frown when disciplines your sub.

And Here's How You Take Someone to Bed

After you master charisma, there is really only one "move" you do to seduce them, which is precisely what the sub wants, since they do not want to be the aggressor.

Tip #9: Always make the conversation about them.

This is true in all human relationships, whether it's BDSM, vanilla sex or even sales. If you want the "customer" to buy, in this case your sub to obey you, you must make EVERYTHING about them and their need.

Talking too much about yourself is pointless because that does not appeal to your sub's ego. Their ego needs to be assuaged and "trained" to their liking. The only thing that matters about your personality is how it affects the subject – your sub.

Tip #10: Be a very good listener.

Sometimes paying attention to what a person says (especially in the negotiation phase) is the best way to become a Master Dom with power over the human mind.

The first part of this obvious: use the person's name. Pay attention to them. Engage them and get their honest thoughts. Empathize with what they're feeling.

The second part is to use the sub's own words to seduce her; borrow their phrasing, their ideas and "mirror" the conversation back at them, getting them to draw closer to you.

Ironically, you will find that the better you are at listening, the less actual research and hard work you have to do when it comes to seducing a sub.

Most subs want to be seduced. So remember your strategic game plan. Make it more about HER and less about you.

We've already talked a great deal about confidence but what does confidence actually look like? That's the theme of our next chapter.

Chapter 3: A Guide to Becoming More Confident as a Dom

Becoming an alpha, Dom, Master or even just a confident male or female in control of others around you SEEMS like a much more difficult process than it really is. Understand that much of human communication is non-verbal. We send messages simply in the way we stand or sit, the way we look at others, our body language and the tone in our voice.

The words that come out, you could say, at least in theory, are of secondary importance. For example, if you were to say "Come to me," and another person were to say, "I desire you to come over here." It's pretty much the same statement. The more effective command won't really be an issue of word usage; just tone of voice and posturing.

Tip #11: Always be alpha by standing up straight, sticking your shoulders out and

holding your stomach in. Your chin should be up.

If you have trouble doing this naturally, exercise more often and make your body become accustomed to this posturing.

The key is to look as tall and alert as possible.

Tip #12: Slow down. Way down from your hyper-talking and nervous persona.

The bottom line is that alphas are not fast-moving unless there is a physical threat or some other reason for more intense movement. Otherwise, they move slowly because slow and deliberate actions boost confidence. If you are a naturally nervous and high-strung person then practice speaking slower, moving slower and mirroring the natural tempo of the sub.

Tip #13: It's not enough to smile – Pay Attention!

Smiling is an excellent move and vital to building trust and friendship as a master seducer of subs. But you can't be constantly happy or jokey and especially not during scenes where you must administer discipline.

Remember the example of The Teacher. The Teacher smiles at first, when he is welcoming his students. But eventually his smile will disappear when he is giving orders or relaying important information. This is naturalism; the ability to give off moods with just your eyes, lips and facial movements. Sometimes the Teacher may even frown or made an angry face as punishment or as warning for the student to obey.

Paying attention to the dynamic of the room and **the mood of the scene** is the most important element.

Tip #14: Win the Staring Contest.

This is such a simple lesson and yet one that a lot of Dom wannabes have trouble with. One of the easiest ways to establish authority is to simply *stare the sub down*. Seems easy enough right? And yet, a lot of people can't handle the intensity of a Staring Contest. It sounds childish and silly but people still do it—and you'll notice the contest happening more often when you're an adult.

It's simply hard-wired into our brains that the more powerful competitor is the one who stares longest. So always try to stare down the sub, or even just random people you meet that give you a funny look. Maybe that look is curiosity or attraction. If you don't stare them down or if you flinch and look away, THEY WIN. You lose. They lose the attraction to you as the alpha.

But wait, isn't staring at people going to creep them out? Actually, it won't, provided you **smile**, nod and generally blink like a normal relaxed person. The only time your stare becomes scary is if you alter the natural shape of your eyes, lose your smile, and never flinch. This "maniacal stare" might serve you well in a scene, but in the negotiation or meeting phase, it's unnecessary. Focus on being friendly and approachable but still alpha. You may be surprised at how often you win these staring contests just by putting forth minimal effort.

If you don't tend to look people in the eye naturally, then work on it. Always dress up to impress when you go out so that you can feel naturally confident and that energy will pass to other people.

Tip #15: Destroy awkwardness at all cost.

You will find that one of the most damaging elements to building your new Alpha Dom persona is awkward energy. And here's the problem. The longer you think about attraction, the worse you get at building it. A shy person's natural inclination is to avoid situations and people that make them nervous. That's a mistake because this fuels your fear and anxiety, while also sending a warning signal to all potential subs that you're not naturally dominant.

Fix this by getting out and meeting everyone you see, and by introducing yourself to whomever you're interested **within seconds** of seeing them for the first time. The immediate follow up to a look, a stare or a glance means everything. If you wait then you communicate fear, or at least disinterest. Neither is advantageous to you. Remember to talk slowly and have some general idea about WHAT thoughts you want to convey; in other words, a strategy of sorts. This prevents nervous energy from building and becoming unbearable.

Tip #16: Take risks.

Remember the billionaire alpha male we talked about? He is a natural born risk taker, and so should you be. Shy guys and subs are the ones who are too afraid to take risks. They must be seduced into releasing their inhibitions. As the teacher, you must help them embrace their wild side. In other words, help them to take risks. If you're too afraid to take risks, by being outgoing, or by saying what you **really** feel (as opposed to the polite, safe conversation we all tend to keep up) then you're never going to convince a sub to take risks herself.

Don't be afraid of anything, including rejection. If you come on too strong, then you can try again later or even analyze what happened and learn from your mistakes. But fearing rejection is only going to hold you back.

Tip #17: Study yourself and learn your strength and weaknesses.

You don't actually have to pretend to be someone you're not. In fact, it's a better idea to become "naturally alpha" or dominant by focusing on your strengths and avoiding competition in areas that you're not skilled in. For example, if you're book smart that's your strength and that's where you gravitate. If you're not naturally witty then avoid trying so hard to be funny during the first meeting. If you're not scientifically well-read, then focus on accentuating your creativity or humor.

Are there certain places where you're just not confident? Grocery stores, bars or clubs, and so on, then avoid them. Are you more comfortable flirting online, in person or in a group? You would come to learn these things about yourself and make an effort to highlight your strengths.

Tip #18: Always expect to be successful.

One of the most de-motivational things in life is trying a new mission knowing you're just going to fail. It's demoralizing. No wonder then that athletes always put so much importance on winning. Because if you go into a contest thinking you've already lost it, the fire is gone. It's the same deal when it comes to alpha Dom confidence.

Expect success. Succeed in all things, even if you must first accomplish little things instead of monumental challenges. Enjoying success helps you visualize future success. And visualizing your desired lifestyle helps you achieve it.

You have to believe that you can win, otherwise you create a self-fulfilling prophecy of failure.

Sounds reasonable so far, right?

But what happens when someone throws you a curve ball? Oh, it will definitely happen! Let's talk about it in the next chapter.

Chapter 4: How to Pass a Sub's Tests

So everything going's along fine. You're feeling confident and your sub appears to be submitting to your authority. All is well. The promise of sex and discipline is intensifying.

And then all of a sudden, the sub does a complete 360 and shatters your confidence. Not fair!

What apparently has happened is that the sub has decided you did not pass one of her tests and so are now unworthy to be a Dom. Why does this happen? What are these tests?

These tests could be anything in terms of words and scenarios. However, all she is really doing is testing your confidence and Dominance factor. She is essentially testing you to see if you show any signs of fear, confusion, or any other form of weakness. If she senses that you're afraid for whatever reason, you're out of the picture.

Her "test" could be a simple question that seems a bit "loaded"; as in, "Gee if I say this she might think I... but if I say this...she might think..."

Or it may just be a total "bitch" move, where the sub does something mean, disrespectful, or cruel.

Usually tests from subs (which are often female in nature but sometimes can be unisex) are:

- Asking a boring question that "filters you out" (usually what you do for work – as if that matters)

- Asking some loaded question that makes you doubt yourself

- When she teases you, mocking you for a laugh (which she pretends is friendly)

- She deliberately insults you (or your Dom personality/scene)

- She friend-zones you, or dismisses your Dom potential

- She flirts with someone else or seems distracted by you

- She starts scaling back and sending negative body language indicating she's lost interest in you

- She disobeys your command or laughs off your training

The question is how are you as the Dom going to react to a blatant test?

Tip #19: Choose your own adventure:

- **(A) Ignore the sub's ridiculous test and press on**

- **(B) Play mind games right back at her and win at all cost**

- **(C) Say something provocative back to her and take a risk**

Each of these reactions has its own advantage and disadvantage.

First, understand that all that is really happening is that the sub is giving you another "test" to determine if you're worthy and a better option than the other Doms she could be seeing. It's a challenge that you must rise to, if you're still interested in her.

Now some Doms will just dismiss a sub that blatantly disrespects them. It's part of their no-tolerance contract. That's up to you.

However, if you think your sub is just being a bad girl (or sissy) and wants to be punished here's what you can do to respond to the test.

1. Ignore the test and continue with the training, adding more discipline. This may be what she wants anyway.

2. Laugh off her test and show that you are not intimidated by her bratty behavior. She has essentially failed to make you nervous and cause you to doubt yourself.

3. Tease her or insult her back.

If she is "abusing you" or "disrespecting you" then you can fire back at her, insulting or provoking her just the same. She may be craving more extremes, and thus will appreciate you upping the ante. Or maybe she just needs to be disciplined once so that she respects your authority.

All that is happening in this scenario is that your sub is trying to throw you off. She's improvising. She's testing you and trying to disqualify you. Don't let her…and make her pay for her disrespect by administering the punishment you see fit (and which of course she likes).

It should be noted that not all subs think alike, just as some women and men react differently. What one person sees as a test may actually be just a genuine curiosity coming from another person.

For example, let's say you're giving your sub a hot sexual scenario. But all of a sudden she criticizes the scene. Not a safe word, just a criticism which seems to be taunting you. You have to use your own judgment to determine if she simply wants something changed or if she is challenging your role as the Dom. If it's the latter you cannot compromise. She knows better than to question your role as the Dom or else she wouldn't be doing a scene in the first place.

The dynamic is also similar during the meeting and negotiation phase. Subs may throw curve balls out to you, and see how you respond to a little conflict. If you are truly confident in your own ability, you won't falter. You'll rise to meet her, slap her down (so to speak) and create an even stronger attraction than before.

It should also be noted that in hardcore BDSM, the dynamic between alpha and submissive is a little more extreme and exaggerated than in "regular dating."

For instance, in regular dating if a woman "tests" a man by asking an interview sort of question, he might laugh off the test by making a joke. Seems appropriate in the context of a first meeting.

However, if you're in the middle of a BDSM scene, then you're not actually supposed to laugh and break concentration. Nor do you want to lose the mood of the scene by laughing off her test. Instead, you would "punish her" instead of just "rising to her challenge." The sub WANTS discipline and any so-called test is done with the sole intention of testing you and hoping that you will escalate the punishment a little higher.

It's the same dynamic as when a student "tests" her teacher, by being bratty or deliberately disobeys a direct order. A strict teacher will not tolerate this "test" and will punish the student with severity. The same is true in the BDSM world—at least if the sub still wants you as her Dom.

If by some chance you upset the sub and fail the test because of your hostility, then it's probably best to just let her go. If she doesn't respect you, and challenges you, and then runs away when you stand up for yourself there is a definite mismatch happening. She really needs to decide at that point whether she's a sub or a Dom and what she actually wants out of this relationship.

If the possibility of losing your sub scares you, then avoid taking risks and avoid escalating the discipline. Instead, speaking honestly with the sub during the after talk session following the scene and discuss how you feel and what she expects you to do.

Punishment, discipline and sex. Where and how does it all come together? How can you recognize the right time to progress a scene into more extreme action? That's the subject of our next chapter.

Chapter 5: Three Hour Foreplay and Aftercare

One of the easiest ways to define BDSM is by the simple description of "three hour foreplay." Most sexual encounters in western civilization end with the formula of very little foreplay, followed by fast, goal-oriented sexual intercourse and release of tension.

This "quickie" style of sex is sometimes preferable, but usually it's a disappointment—especially if it becomes a routine. Sex is supposed to be an art form that is dense with psychological stimulation and eroticism.

As we've already discussed, BDSM can be so intense that it doesn't even require penetration, oral sex or any genital touching. Some people literally just want to be spanked or hurt and do not want to be sexually fulfilled.

This could be because they consider the spanking the most exciting part of the session, or it could be because they don't consider consensual spanking as actual sex. Whatever the sub's reasoning, it is a legitimate consideration.

In BDSM, foreplay is a must. And in the case of non-sexual domination, (spanking, injury, punishment, constraints, etc.) foreplay to the non-penetrative act is STILL foreplay. The reason being that most of this foreplay is mental.

It's true you may incorporate some physical maneuvers into the foreplay or the punishment but the entire scene begins as a mental / emotional experience that triggers the sense of erotic fulfillment.

If you were to ask a typical woman, she might tell you that 10-15 minutes of foreplay is good, and you would probably get an even smaller count from a man.

However, in BDSM, foreplay is always much longer because it involves altering the mental state of the sub for greater orgasmic or cathartic enhancement.

So yes, do plan on devoting at least an hour if not longer to building anticipation for the experience. If you really want to be a good Dom then make it a three hour experience.

Take one hour to prepare the sub and speak frankly and another hour devoted to punishment and training, and then an hour devoted to the aftercare. You could even have three hours' worth of punishment and sexual foreplay if desired…

The only issue is, if you want sex or discipline to last that long, you must pace yourself.

Tip #20: A Dom should choreograph a scene based on his imagination, the sub's contract, and a reasonable assessment of the physical abilities of the sub.

For one thing, you have to consider the physical limitations of three-hour four play. Both men and women, and particularly men who have a longer refractory period after ejaculation, must take frequent breaks. Men usually cannot hold an erection for hours on end, and cock-rings that force hard erections are typically dangerous if worn for an extended period of time.

Therefore, the man must become accustomed to the routine of enjoying his erection, letting it fall back to a lesser level of excitement, and then grow again. This pattern repeats itself. Women may also wish to have a break in between orgasms.

If you are going for the "subspace trance" (discussed in this book later on) then you also have to take frequent breaks after an intense series of punishment and pain, or else you might accidentally hurt the sub beyond what was agreed upon.

Remember that in BDSM, the intent is not necessarily orgasm but triggering pain so as to release feel-good endorphins, along with intensely erotic or taboo scenes that manipulate the sub's emotions. The goal is to punish the sub in increments of about 10-20 minutes and then wait for the good pain killing chemicals to come in, bringing the sub into subspace.

If you go beyond peripheral pain and consistently increase the pain threshold, eventually you will set the sub into a "fight or flight" state of mind and release adrenaline, which is another phase. This is another period of rest that may require some recovery time. The Dom continues "training" during these feel-good subspace moments, namely by talking and giving directions to the sub. However, the pain temporarily stops—for approximately 5-10 minutes—before picking back up and starting the cycle again.

Naturally, new subs or subs that just met you, are not going to want long and intensive sessions of subspace trance. You have to work your way up to a deeper level of trust by starting slow and steadily progressing to the top of the scale.

Tip #21: Follow the punishment formula for subspace, including the breaks.

Pain and pleasure together will trigger activity from the sympathetic nervous system; this includes releasing epinephrine from the adrenal glands, as well as endorphins and enkephalins.

In practical terms, this is almost a morphine like high, since the chemicals are released into the blood stream, and thus not only provide pleasure and numbing but also INCREASES THE PAIN TOLERANCE. Increasing the pain tolerance allows for even greater enhancement.

The deeper the sub goes into the state, by experiencing more pain, the more she will actually become numb, or even incoherent as if high on drugs. You cannot necessarily gauge by timing schedule alone—you must watch your sub and make sure that she is not being pushed beyond what she can bear.

Bear in mind that the euphoric subspace state can last literally hours or even days. At some point you must stop. Subspace can also affect the sub's ability to make rational decisions, hence, the need for intensive aftercare.

Aftercare is not part of foreplay really, but it's a must—at least an hour is recommended if your sub is new and if the experience reaches a high level of intensity.

The sub may not even want to take a break—they may think they can handle more than they actually can. But keep in mind these are very forbidden desires they are just now learning; they are also experiencing a new kind of raw, emotive form of communication, playing with their ego and id. This level of excitement literally requires some "coming down" time. There is also a profound mental effect going on here, as the sub confronts complex psychological issues related to childhood, childhood discipline, guilt, fear and so on.

So just remember that as much as effort as you put into three-hour foreplay, it is a full experience and one that requires a long-term approach.

You may be surprised to know that even Tops and Doms can experience the "Drop" from subspace, and ending the session abruptly without aftercare only seems to make it worse. This drop could even lead to depression or hangover like symptoms.

Preparing the Sub as Part of Foreplay

If you really want to give your sub an affair to remember, the goal is to extend the pre-touching and pre-punishing psychological foreplay for as long as possible. Now you may be thinking, "Well I can discipline her good for a whole ten minutes before the punishment starts…that's about enough, right?"

The sub ultimately decides how long she wants foreplay and punishment, but you're usually encouraged to extend the psychological foreplay for a longer period of time, as this will make the climax more intense, and maybe without the need for excessive body stimulation.

BDSM is largely about the uneven power dynamic and discipline, and the physical pain-pleasure delivery is second. Therefore, one of the best ways to extend psychological foreplay is to spend time emphasizing the power that the Dom wields over the sub.

Tip #22: Choose the right position for a sub so that she can feel your power.

This involves choosing a "slave position" for punishment. These positions are meant so that the Dom can enable the slave to better serve and please him and accept training.

The position will accomplish each of the following:

1. Submission to the Dom

2. Better concentration so she will obey commands

3. Establishing a feel of helplessness and total reliance on the sub

4. An ideal punishment for discipline, such as spanking

5. An easy position for examining the sub's body

6. Easy sexual access (even if sex is not requested)

7. Allows the slave to learn patience and endurance

8. Established a default position for a "controlled behavior"

Number eight simply means that the sub should be trained according to a plan and a scene that has a beginning, middle and end. In order for the peaks to stand out, a "controlled behavior" should be established to contrast the peaks of excitement, which involve more radical body contact or movement. So start with something simple, like a blindfold, and then move slowly into more drastic physical constraints.

You can also train your sub to take a controlled / default position, when you haven't given any specific orders. This is known as *parking your sub*. Assigning a **Teaching Word** is the way of creating a verbal command that demands attention and a standard position of submission.

Part of total dominance and demanding complete submission requires inspection of the sub's body, since this creates trust while also destroying all sense of privacy. When you have a sub there should be no physical privacy. Not only for training purposes but also so you as the responsible one can check for any bruises, infections or other potential problems.

Slaves or subs can become "living art" to the Master so there is no "impossible" position, if the Dom and sub are in agreement.

Positions Commonly Used

- **Attention**: The sub keeps her feet and ankles together, arms at the side and back straight. It's mimicking standard military positioning.

- **Assume**: This position has the sub standing behind and to the left of the Dom, usually on the floor, sitting on her lower legs, as this tends to be easier on the legs than kneeling for long periods of time.

- **Auction**: Slave standing with legs apart and arms stretched out diagonally to face the crowd and present their body.

- **Crawl / Fetch**: Sending a slave to pick up an object, usually on her knees and palms. She is usually ordered to pick up objects with her mouth. An alternative version of this position is "Table" when the slave holds her head down in shame while on all fours. The Dom may even use her body as furniture.

- **Come**: A standing position but with the face down and arms and legs controlled, not sticking out.

- **Present**: Face down with arms stretched over the sub's head, and the wrists and ankles crossed in a sort of symbolic constraint.

- **Following**: Always four steps to the back and left of the Dom, when he is walking. If the Dom wishes to speak, the slave walks to his right.

- **Back**: When sitting on her back the sub should have her legs together and arms to her side.

- **Display**: Like a police control position, the sub will lock her fingers behind her head and stand up straight, displaying their body and showing surrender. She can be on knees or standing for this one.

- **Parade Rest**: This position involves willful constraint, as the sub must spread her feet widely apart and put her arms behind her back, with one hand in the other towards her lower back.

- **Face Down / Worship**: She moves from a standing position into a face down position, but with a slow presentation to her Dom / Audience. Her knees should be kept under her chest and her head prostrated to the floor. Her arms would be extended straight, palms down, and by her head.

- **Go to**: A sub is sent to a location in the house or dungeon to await further instruction. She may be asked to stick her nose in the corner, as if time out for adults.

- **Surrender**: The sub lies with her face to the ground, her ankles crossed and arms over her head with wrists crossed—as if tied up.

- **Cross**: This is a position of humility, with the arms out in a cross position, with legs parted wide, and either lying face down or on her back.

- **Whipping Position**: She can be standing or kneeing for this. The sub leans against a surface and exposes her back and butt for punishment. If she is kneeling, she presents herself in the air. She will protect her hands and neck by shielding them underneath her body.

- **Indian Style**: On the floor, the sub bends her knees and spreads her legs slightly, with her ankles crossed. She rests her palms on her knees. The subs hands may also be turned in the opposite, with the palms up or out, indicating that she is learning and opening her mind to the sub's teachings.

- **Genital Inspection**: Just like an exam position, except that the sub spreads her vaginal lips or anus for thorough inspection.

- **Punishment Position**: Standing position, one that seems like something you might find on an exercise video. She bends over and grabs her legs with her hands behind her calves. Her legs are typically spread for presentation. This is an ideal position for spanking, but in contrast to the more comfortable position of leaning on a surface on arching her back.

- **Bondage**: In addition to the cross position, often used with bedroom restraints, the default bondage position is when the sub is made to lay on her back with her head turned to one side, with her hands in the small of her back and legs crossed at the ankle. She may be tied with a rope or be ordered to get into this position so that she can be tied.

A sub should beware of:

- Slouching (back should be kept straight)

- Turning Her Back, a sign of disrespect, since a sub is not supposed to turn her back while in session

- Face should be down, or face up with eyes down. Eye contact with the Dom is usually requested, since the sub looking at him without permission is considered aggressive.

Classwork and Homework

One of the best ways to make foreplay last longer is to start viewing your sessions more like a curriculum than a sex scene. For instance, you have the plans of action written beforehand, which is based on the sub's own contract and requests. Now it's time to figure out what points are important for the sub to learn and what can be learned via "homework". That's right, you can put your sub to work outside of the scene.

For instance, some Doms order their subs to work out at the gym or to groom themselves in a certain way, preparing for their next session well in advance. This is a way for the sub to demonstrate her loyalty while also making the foreplay last longer.

Homework assignments can be anything including:

- Showering and shaving

- Hairstyling and makeup requests

- Specifics sets of clothing or having the sub ask the Dom for permission to wear something she chooses

- Doing chores in said clothing

- Cooking and cleaning

- Practice positions or sexual behaviors at home to get better at them

- Take photographs

- Wearing chastity belts to assure the sub's fidelity

Examples of classwork are more intensive and may involve:

- Getting the sub to change into positions of the Master's choosing; teaching them to remember these positions

- Shaming, or "branding" of the sub via marker, body piercing or tattooing

- Programming the slave to say something specific or feel a certain way, based on punishment

- Disciplining, or for more intense play, degrading the sub in a previously negotiated way

- Being tied up or made to wear sex furniture or use sex toys

- Public humiliation, making the sub go out in public still submitting to his commands

- Reprogramming her speech patterns, her behavior and her appearance

- Getting the sub to act like an animal

Tip #23: The work you give your sub to do are really just a way to show that you are an attentive Dom, intent on teaching her important points—all of which contribute to transforming her into the sub / slave she wants to become.

More on this later. Remember though, that if you don't have a strategy and no classwork or homework, the sub may feel underwhelmed, as if she's not really getting any "training" out of the relationship – just massaging your own ego.

The sub will be patient but you have to be teaching her something and you have to remind her what she is teaching. This means…

Tip #24: Tell your sub what you are teaching her.

The sub may miss the more subtle points you are trying to convey unless you make it very explicit what you are doing.

For example, if you're training her to be more self-confident and sexual, then are you giving her dialog to say? Are you teaching her why she should become more self-confident and what parts of her body are arousing? Are you consistently talking to her and reprogramming her thoughts to think more positively about her appearance and sexual desires? Homework could be making her work out or dress in a certain way. Classwork with you, may involve having sex with her, or making her speak her desires aloud.

Punishment is the part that usually has a limited time frame, since as we discussed you must be careful not to overtax her body and over-punish or injure her in the heat of the moment.

In terms of organizing a curriculum punishment, know that punishment must always be accompanied by an explanation, or else it just makes you a sadist. For instance, if she is disobedient, if she is contrary, or if she forgets to do her assigned homework, that is a good reason to administer punishment. That way, her subconscious mind learns that it's less stressful to obey you.

The punishment should be something that she is slightly uncomfortable with, but that she still allows for in the contract you make. This way, you are still disciplining her by delivering an unfavorable reaction to specific behaviors. This reprograms the mind to seek out positive behavior. So you must learn what makes her uncomfortable (differentiated from what terrifies her, which you never do) and then do it as a means of punishment.

If she craves punishment, then you can schedule punishment sessions based on missed homework or for committing transgressions behind your back. You assume she did so, and so punish her for all the bad stuff you missed.

Even if it seems "unfair" there is still a logic to it. She is learning that bad behavior results in something she doesn't necessarily like – something that even slightly hurts.

On the other hand, all classwork and evidence of completed homework should result in something she really does like and feels excited by. If she is a masochist and loves spanking, then spanking would be a reward. You would find another means of punishing her, whether it's withholding, emotional discipline, restraint, and so on.

Therefore...

Tip #25: Write down in your own private notes what she likes and dislikes and plan a curriculum of:

- What she wants to feel (her immediate needs)

- What she needs to learn (long-term happiness)

- What system of reward will keep her motivated

- What system of punishment will keep her honest

- How you will schedule each session, teaching one point at a time.

This approach may require that you create a finite timeline, rather than an ongoing relationship. If it works, then that's a good thing. After all, you're doing this for her, not for your own pleasure. If you need your ego stroked so badly that you would keep a sub eternally reliant on you rather than help teach her something valuable, then it's time for you to become the sub. Because the sub is the one with the issues to work out. Not the Dom.

Now, granted, some subs WANT to become reliant on a Dom for an indefinite period of time. This is when they officially become a slave, someone who constantly craves the presence of their Master. Typically the sub wants a limited relationship. Slaves will be indefinitely attached to their master. Of course, since this is an ongoing relationship, the slave and the Master both may develop interests and desires outside the exclusive relationship, which explains the next section…

The More the Merrier

Although not all subs want multiple Doms, some do. At some point you may find that bringing in additional subs or Doms in order to train your sub may be effective. This works in teaching, as the presence of another educator is always more powerful. The same is true in BDSM lifestyle.

Doms may order their sub/slave to service other Doms, sexually or otherwise, or may combine their efforts with another slave. The question is, what's the point of bringing in all these other people?

It has to be related to the curriculum. If the main intention is to get the sub to become more uninhibited with sex, then it's easy to see why making her service other men would be either reward or punishment, depending on how she is responding to the curriculum. However, a common misconception is that all subs are just desiring humiliation and sluthood.

That's not necessarily the case. Some subs may not want sex at all, while others might allow some form of sexual contact—but not just anything. Some subs really do want a some kind of therapy from the experience, and not just a good time. See Chapter for 9 for more on this.

We have previously stated in this book series that new Doms ought to seek out experience by being trained by other Doms. It is an option you have to become a sub first, to experience how the other side lives, and we talk about this a little bit later. However, this is not a rule.

Some Doms only want to be Doms and rather than become subs, they simply mentor with other Doms. So...

Tip #26: Find another Dom in your local area and accompany him on one of his sub training sessions.

It's great to see an experienced Dom in action, to see how the job is done in real life and in real time. You can analyze how he performs, how he controls his voice and body and how he develops the curriculum of the training. You can compare how his example relates to the text you've read thus far. Textbook knowledge will give you an intellectual advantage. But watching it in person, and following the other Dom's lead when he lets you discipline or train his sub, will give you more confidence and more emotional understanding of how to set up a scene on your own.

Doms who are secure in their power and confidence will not be threatened by you. They will let you accompany them on a training session, provided you are friendly, honest and upfront about what you want. Always respect the elder Dom's property, methods and opinions. If you disagree with something he thinks or says, then learn from it. There's no need to be a jerk and start correcting him. He may deal with his sub in a different way than you would and if you don't like it, find your own sub and create your own superior system.

Many new Doms are confused as to whether subs want sex or just punishment and discipline. We've devoted a whole chapter to understanding the many ways in which we enjoy intimacy with our submissive partners.

Chapter 6: How Many Ways Are There to Enjoy Intimacy?

It's important to separate the idea of sex from intimacy. Sex is either procreation (intercourse that could result in pregnancy if factors are right) or it is for release.

Most sexual encounters are all about attraction and release. Much of what we learn about sex from the movies teaches us that sex is goal oriented and that it only has to last several intense moments. Rough foreplay followed by sexual penetration and release.

However, this modern and corrupted view of sex strips the act of all sensuality and intimacy. In Eastern civilization, sexuality has always been connecting with intimacy, sensual response and even religious and deeply spiritual experiences. Tantric sex, for example, uses religious symbols to help its practicing lovers reach higher levels of orgasm, awareness and connectivity to their partner, the universe and the deities up above.

It's also no coincidence that Tantric sex and the Americanized version of it, known clinically as Sensate Focus, focuses on eliminating the goal of sex. This is why in BDSM, we're going to do the same thing...

Tip #27: Stop thinking of sex or BDSM play as a penis/vagina encounter.

In fact, just eliminate that option altogether for the time being. Now focus on what ELSE you can do, until you become good at it.

By the time you come up with new and creative methods of foreplay and sexual teasing, your sub may actually crave genital touching or penetration, and then if you want, you can give it to her as a reward for good behavior. However, depriving her and yourself of the simple sex act is one of the best ways to up your game and deliver a more sensual experience.

Let's break down Intimacy into 11 different stages, all of which are options to consider in your overall curriculum. You may even want to re-do some stages, just to make sure the sub learns. In class, your students may need to go over a chapter multiple times to learn and remember the information. In the same like manner, it may actually take several sessions to teach one important point to your sub.

Stage 1: Seduction and Dominance

This is the part where you must first seduce the sub, offering her a lesson in BDSM. Then, your focus is in building trust and gaining her complete trust and obedience. She must find your dominance arousing or else there will be no reason to submit.

This is usually the stage where the most verbal play and mind games are used. You are breaking down her opposition to submitting to you. This is when she tests you and when you prove yourself as an alpha male who is in control of yourself and in control of all your relationships.

Common Techniques

- Flirting and teasing

- Offering the commodity of your Dom experience

- Mirroring her thoughts, words and body language

- Demonstrating power and control, essentially telling her what to do casually (as in volunteering places you could go together – taking control of the date)

- Manipulating emotional peaks (avoiding normal date behavior and instead stimulating her emotions through conflict or intriguing conversation)

Stage 2: Building Suspense and Anticipation

This flirting and mental engagement heightens the sensual interest for your training. It's important to note that the sub should actually be expecting a lot more than "just sex"; you are offering a teaching experience, which is much more promising than just ordinary sex.

Not only is this the stage where you make the offer to train your sub (definitely letting them know you are in the lifestyle), but you must also let her know that it will require a contract. This lets her know that you are serious about this BDSM relationship and that you take consent seriously.

Common Techniques

- The **contract** is a great way to build anticipation. Not only does it make clear all your intentions, and get the all-important CONSENT from her--but it also gives you a great glimpse into her mind, making it easier to develop discipline and punishment unique to her character. Focus on what she likes, what she is slightly afraid of, and definitely avoid whatever she forbids. Just making this contract (and all the unknowns of what you will do to her) will make her curious and excited to be experimenting in the lifestyle.

- **Role Playing** is another technique of sensuality that can very easily become eroticism. You assume a character as does she, which relieves you of all responsibilities of being the "ethical you." You can experiment more, do things that are uncharacteristic of your usual ID, and take risks. Of course, you as the safe Dom are guiding her in the role play, keeping her safe. But the role play game is a great way to stimulate her mind before physical action.

Stage 3: Making Her Submit

One of the most important forms of foreplay or "sensuality" (not just sex) is the process of having the sub prove her submission to you. Removing her clothes and getting into proper position is one major step because it involves the loss of her power, and presenting herself to you to control.

Common Techniques

- Making her take off her clothes

- Making her take off your clothes

- Ordering her to act like an animal

- Ordering her to get into proper position

- Making her do chores

Stage 4: Touching

In sex, kissing is often a prelude to foreplay and intercourse. Not all subs will desire kissing, since this action may mean love to them. However, some may just consider kissing another form of touching. Therefore, all non-genital touching would be included in physical sensual foreplay; that is stimulating the person's body.

Whereas in other forms of sensuality/sex, touching may be a joyful experience, in BDSM it is usually more about gaining control and demonstrating to the sub that you have full power. You want to know her body and let her know that it is no longer hers to work with but yours. You are going to mold her body and mind into the kind of person she wants to be, and that you can make her.

Common Techniques

- Caressing her body

- Massaging her body (deeper and harder strokes)

- Playing with her body for your own amusement

- Experimenting to see where her erogenous zones are and where she is most sensitive

Stage 5: Genital or Breast Touching

Again, this may or may not be requested. But genital touching without penetration is the next stage, since this causes direct sexual arousal. This may even be a form of reward-based pleasure that you give the sub for good behavior.

What is different about BDSM genital touching and regular intercourse is that you usually don't give the sub direct penetration. This is because intercourse could cause you to lose control over yourself and the session. But your entire focus is in controlling the sub and making her feel what she needs to feel. Therefore, it's highly advised that you not penetrate or ejaculate unless it's some type of reward/punishment behavior at the end of the session. It's simply too goal-oriented and you have far too much to do in training than to limit yourself.

Common Techniques

- Clitoral stimulation
- G-spot stimulation
- A-spot or Deep Spot stimulation

- Breast stimulation

- Oral sex, anal sex, breast sex, handjobs, footjobs or fetishism

- Prostate massage (for dominated men, involving a G-spot equivalent in males located 2-3 inches inside the anus)

Stage 6: Establishing Rules and Discipline

This is essential as the entire scene is pointless without the communication of the rules and discipline. Discipline IS a form of sensuality all its own and it is so intense that sexual intercourse, or even genital touching, may not be required after administering discipline and punishment.

This is the stage where she stops thinking and begins feeling. She is no longer constrained by ego, conscience or resistance. You have broken down her resistance through consensual submission. Now it's time to get rid of her conscious thought by telling her exactly what to do, and how the said action is going to make her feel.

After you spend some time reprogramming her mind to feel and obey, she will find it easier to stop thinking and just follow orders. She will enjoy the catharsis of not having to think or rationalize anything. She will simply be.

Common Techniques

- Establishing Slave protocol when the session begins; positions, clothes, etc.

- Interrogating the sub and asking invasive questions

- Making the sub answer honestly, even unflattering or inappropriate questions

- Humiliating the sub in pre-approved ways

- Explaining why what she does or thinks is wrong and needs to be changed

- Explaining to the sub who you want to turn her into – a role model

- Removing freedoms or giving the sub obligations

- Giving homework assignments to keep her mind occupied

- Making her into a "perfect woman"
- Treat her as a pet, one with no rights except to be coddled and loved

Stage 7: Making It Hurt

Punishment is what she fears (though she doesn't forbid it) and so when she submits to it, she will experience a rush of endorphins and eventually adrenaline, depending on how hard to push her.

As we discussed previously, you build up to higher thresholds of pain for greater pleasure-pain peaks. Punishment is inherently part of discipline. Without the threat of punishment, she will not learn how important obedience is.

She must also first experience pain to appreciate pleasure. She will only reach greater rewards (not to mention higher emotional peaks because of the adrenaline rush) if she submits to pain first.

It's true that not all subs will want the same type of pain, so you do have to research your assignment carefully. However, this part of your curriculum is always the planned out and the most complex.

Common Techniques

- Spanking with hand, belt, whip or flogger

- Using restraints; rope, handcuffs, leather, fabric

- Hot / Cold play with candles and ice

- Degradation and name calling or public humiliation

- Performing uncharacteristic or rough sexual acts

- Using clamps on genitals and breasts

Piercing or tattooing

Stage 8: Making Sure She Learns

Making sure she learns is part of the in-scene communication process. What good is teaching your student if you don't test them to see proof of their comprehension?

Same thing with BDSM – you review sessions with your sub in scene, asking her questions while "in character", and then out of character during the aftercare. Then, she will tell you what she wants to see more of and what you could change to improve.

Communication IS sensual and it is a form of building intimacy with another person. Talking can be erotic and therapeutic. And sensuality is all about communicating your desires to your sub and listening to hers.

Common Techniques

- In Session: Asking for yes or no questions

- In Session: Calling herself a degrading name or describing her own flaws

- In Session: Admitting what she's done wrong

- In Session: Explaining to her how her normal thinking process and typical behavior is wrong and must be corrected

- Aftercare: Asking for feedback

- Aftercare: Asking for feelings, and if anything made her too uncomfortable

- Aftercare: Compared to other experiences
- Aftercare: What she would like to try in future sessions

Stage 9: Aftercare

The aftercare period also involves the famous "Cuddling" stage, that most people do practice after regular sex, but are never really sure why. A lot of men are, frankly, afraid of the cuddling stage and prefer to leave as quickly as possible.

Here's what's going on: when you cuddle mindlessly, you just create a comfortable environment. When you cuddle after punishment and training, you create a system of nurturing.

The sub will feel light-headed, maybe even slightly "drugged" if the endorphin and adrenaline rush is high; therefore, they will want nurturing and comfort in order to return to the real world. This helps to build trust and your authority as a teacher.

Common Techniques

- Caressing

- Holding

- Whispering or talking, saying warm and comforting things

- Reprogramming her mind with kind affirmations of the new personality you and she are striving for

- Creating pleasant visuals of the person she wants to become

- Getting her to talk and explain how she feels

- Hugging and kissing her if she cries

- Describing happy thoughts and her happy future (becoming the new personality)

Stage 10: Building Anticipation for Next Time

The sub must feel compelled to come back. If you do the aftercare and plan effectively for a long-term series of sessions, she will want to come back.

Completing a scene and aftercare session requires that you leave the sub with a parting thought. Usually, it's telling them what to expect for the next session, as well as homework.

The teaching process, the assigning of work to do, and the obligation you give the sub is part of the sensual process.

Common Techniques

- Telling her what punishments or rewards the next session will involve

- Explaining something about history, culture or science that relates to her discipline

- Leaving her with a question or a statement to think about

- Giving her homework

- Making her wear a chastity belt

Stage 11: The Nirvana Stage

Many Doms and subs will brag that they, or others they know, have reached a so-called hallucinogenic stage of total devotion and pleasure—a 10 on the scale of climax, which can be achieved through spankings, or sexual stimulation, or some other intensive form of pleasure. We'll explore that in Chapter 8. However, suffice it to say, reaching new emotional and mental states of mind—altered states with your partner—is a great way to transcend regular sex and find a brand new way to experience sensuality.

For the next chapter, let's focus on how to choreograph a session and create a curriculum that trains your sub effectively.

Chapter 7: Live Like a Sub to Discipline Like a Dom

There are really only two ways to learn how to be an excellent Dom – training as a sub or training as an Assistant Dom. It's not always easy to find a Dom that's willing to take you under his wing, best rest assured if you ask nicely and respect the Dom's rules, you can find one in your local BDSM community. Fetlife is a good place to search for members and it's free. Some Doms may even be married men who enjoy showcasing their sub wives, so it's not as hard as you think to find a mentoring Dom.

However, if you have the guts to try it, learning to be a better Dom by becoming a sub first is another way to master the discipline. Becoming a sub first teaches you:

- How the session works and how the Dom leads

- How a sub is supposed to respond (Which you can use in building your own scenes later)

- How toys work and how much they can hurt

- How much pain you can take and how it affects your body

- How to treat other Doms and subs and develop a good reputation

Frankly, experiencing BDSM as the sub is more enjoyable than being the Dom at times, since you're actually more focused on receiving pain and pleasure, and less on worrying about your performance.

The Dom instructs the sub what to do and how to feel. The Dom can also tell the sub what he or she is doing wrong. Some Doms actually stay subs for the people they like, but graduate to becoming a Dom for new subs they meet. There is no set hierarchy. There is no obligation for you to stop being a sub and only being a Dom. This is why *Switches* are fairly popular in the BDSM community, since they are always ready to have a good time, whether on top or on bottom.

And as we've said before, don't believe that subs are weak by nature. Not only are subs in control, but some slaves out there in the BDSM world are far more cruel and demanding than even Master/Doms. Their Master simply lets them dominate other subs and enjoys it. There's really no rules here, so you DO have to...

Tip #28: Find a series of Dom/sub experiences that teaches you about the lifestyle and about yourself.

Here are 5 scenarios you might think about trying:

1. Going to a BDSM club or event where you can meet people

2. Take part in a public exhibition where you punish a willing Sub

3. Arranging to meet a Dom who will introduce you to his sub spouse

4. Arranging to meet a Dom who will become your Sub, teaching you how the sub behaves

5. Watching a Dom and sub group play, in an exhibition or multi-partner encounter

Tip #29: Always stay for the aftercare and ask questions of both the Dom and sub to see what their motivation was, and why they chose a particular discipline or action.

You can also interview Doms and subs off-duty, who will give you additional insight into in-person psychology that you just can't learn from text alone.

The Six Subs You Meet

By now, you understand the lifestyle and once you go to a BDSM club, you're going to get a good idea of how the in-person experience feels like. So let's review the most common TYPES of Doms and subs you meet out there in the BDSM community. While these are clichés and stereotypes, they are typically true of a large portion of the population, so keep this in mind.

1. The Giggly Girl

She wants to be a little girl. She wants a daddy figure. She is also very clingy and jealous of other subs. Oftentimes has low self-esteem.

2. The Rebel

There are definitely subs that just want to test you—and some want to be "tamed" meaning they will rebel unless you punish them harshly. They are very alpha when you meet them, even if they are subs. They need a STRONG Dom to break their spirit and turn them into submissive girls. The downside is she does become bored quickly and is not necessarily a long-term thing.

3. The Sensitive SAM

The SAM (Smart Assed Masochists) is a surprisingly smart and acid-tongued type of sub, who makes it a little hard on you at first. However, they are ultimately playful and this is just their way of communicating. You will find that they usually don't want a lot of punishment. Just strong discipline, usually through words, is typically enough to control them. They are highly sensitive, even if slightly aggressive, and do not ultimately want to upset their Dom.

4. The Anti-Sub

The Anti-Sub has already been claimed by someone else and enjoys challenging Doms for the hell of it, just to make them doubt themselves. They are only submissive to their partner and thus, the only way to control them is to get their partner involved. There are also degrees of Anti-Subs. One of which is the Dom-worshiping sub who seems extremely devoted to their master, almost to the point of obsession.

5. The Perfect Slave

Very committed and usually willing to do or endure anything, but with a bit of an ego. They are really good at what they do, but they oftentimes overstep their bounds and forget the whole point of submission.

6. The True Submissive

The true submissive is not really "perfect" but actually submissive to the Dom, and puts their Dom's wishes and desires above that of her own needs, wants and ego. She is willing to do anything but expects a Dom who truly understands the psychology of dominance. She is typically younger, inexperienced and looking to be taught. She is often shy. Some speculate that all Bad subs start off as the True Submissive but are corrupted by poor quality Doms and become one of the subs listed above.

Common Mistakes Made by Dums (Not Doms!)

The ideal Dom is YOU! Someone who understands the textbook psychology of BDSM and has also sought out in-person experience under sub or Dom training from another person. He is patient, and focused on the needs and contractual obligations of the sub. Therefore, a good sub is only trying to please the Dom and a good Dom is only trying to please the sub and things work out perfectly.

However, there are bad Doms out there. Rather than explaining the most common mistakes Dom make, let's consider the types of imposter Doms that subs are trying to avoid.

1. The Psycho Dom

Tries so hard to be "dominant" without understanding technique he's just an abusive jerk.

2. The Toy Master

Sort of knows what he's doing, but is mostly just interested in showing off his new BDSM toys. Doesn't quite the get the nuances.

3. The Horny Guy

Total imposter, just wants to have sex. Doesn't understand anything about BDSM except that he's impersonating some billionaire guy. Often switches from Dom to sub in desperation.

4. The Slut Dom

Dom sluts are Doms that seek out new subs frequently, and is not a very committed type of teacher.

5. The Control Freak

Some subs may like him, but not all will. He is so dominant he's almost unbearable to play with. He stalks his sub, micromanages her, is invasive and doesn't respect boundaries. He may be dangerous, so tread carefully if you're a sub seeking Dom training.

6. The Married Dom

Make sure married Doms are in an open relationship. Many Doms are married but ultimately are omegas, not alphas, since they are keeping secrets from their wife and have limited time to play.

7. The Clueless Dom

He claims he's a Dom but has no idea what he's doing. He's without a curriculum, without a game plan, and barely understands the process of negotiation and the contract. He's just not ready for primetime yet.

8. The Sissy Dom

For lack of a better term…the Sissy Dom is confused. He's not actually a switcher, he just wants to be a Dom, even though he's only really good at being a sub. He tries hard, but doesn't seem to understand the psychology of discipline.

There are other types of Doms, such as Mommy or Daddy Doms who enjoy disciplining surrogate children, sadists who only want to inflict pain, and also "Lesser Gods" which just want to be worshiped. Farmers are Doms who specialize in collecting slaves, treating them like animals and may actually want to just hand them over to someone else.

Be sure that you are the Alpha Billionaire Dom, and not too much of a niche specialist. The only way to enjoy this community is to be an adaptable Dom who knows what he's doing and desires to please a sub.

Tip #30: Get to know your partner (whether a Dom or sub) and ask them plenty of interview questions to gauge how much they understand about the psychology of what they are doing in their role.

Subs don't have to know as much about this, but Doms really have to be instructed in the finer arts of seduction, training and discipline. Otherwise, you can see through them quickly.

Putting on the Mind of Your Partner

Tip #31: If you want to become a sub for training purposes, be honest with yourself

and determine what you want from a Dom and what you want to feel.

This involves admitting your fetishes, your taboos, and you're "never will" items that are off limits. Creating one of these forms is essential to understanding what you want to hear from a sub.

So an example Sub Contract might be something like:

- I have issues with discipline because of my strict upbringing

- I desire to dominated by someone strict, who will pleasure and punish me

- I am a little nervous about spankings and being tied up. But the idea does also turn me on.

- I am attracted to taboos of parental sexual discipline.

- I do NOT want any anal penetration or being called degrading names.

Based on a contract like this, the Dom would put together a curriculum for the slave or sub based on the wishes and requests. Like:

- Week 1: Establish my role as a surrogate parent. Make the sub respect my authority.

- Week 2: Establish a system of rules on what the sub does with his life. The sub will be given chores and homework to do. Failure to do them will result in punishment.

- Week 3: The sub is becoming too comfortable. Must break the sub's spirit in order for punishment to be effective. Invent new rules. Punish for unseen instances.

- Week 4: Make the sub beg and apologize for breaking the rules. Tie up and punish with tickle torture and spanking. Then make the sub apologized. Ground the sub for disrespect and remove privileges. If she responds obediently, give her sexual reward.

As you can see, many of these exercises were based on what the sub was doing during training. If she was losing respect for the Dom, then the sub would have to be punished and their spirit broken down until a humbler attitude appeared. The sub explored the taboos carefully, not all at once and incorporated them into a system of reward and discipline.

This is the best reason to experience BDSM play as a sub—because it gives you experience in writing contracts, seeing live sessions, and aftercare. The negotiation and aftercare would also be detailed in curriculum since this is just as important. For example:

Week 1:

Negotiation: Explain that I will be punishing and rewarding. Review taboos and forbidden acts. Explain to my sub that I will not allow rebellion or the relationship is over.

Aftercare: Cuddle the sub after punishment, treating them like as a surrogate child, letting them know that they are still loved.

Aftermath Talk: Discuss what worked and what didn't. What the sub wants to see more of and less of.

Tip #32: Putting yourself in your sub's mind is the best thing you can do in preparing to be a Dom.

Therefore, you must study your sub through:

- Informal Conversation (Take mental notes of what they seem to want)

- By contract (What they explicitly say they want)

- How responsive they are to my ideas based on body language and tone of voice

- By direct suggestion during negotiation

- Discussion in the aftercare dialog

How to Draw Out a Shy Sub

What about subs who really don't know what they want but who seem intrigued at your offer to teach them? There are subs that may test you a little bit, perhaps unintentionally, but they do manage to make it hard on you, since they don't reveal much about their kinks.

Maybe they're just too vanilla to realize that they have kinks. If this is the case then take this three-pronged approach:

Tip #33: Ask them questions about their life, their upbringing and their values in life.

Most people will admit what these are. Use this information to determine what they "secretly want."

For example, if they say they had parents who used corporal punishment growing up, they probably are attracted to spankings. If they were very close to their opposite sex parent, they may have a surrogate parent kink and crave discipline. If they mention an ex-girlfriend or boyfriend they probably still have baggage from that. Find out the "villain" role of this sub's life and assume it, whether it's a strict parent, a boss, an ex, or what have you.

You can also study "market research" and find out what other subs say turns them on and ask your sub if they would be opposed to trying something like that. It is best to ask outright rather than just introducing something foreign into the relationship. When in doubt always ask. Your sub might appreciate you coming up with new and unusual ideas.

We've written a lot thus far about putting your partner into trance. And if you are having trouble bringing your sub to climax, you may be wondering what you're doing wrong. This is the focus of Chapter 8.

Chapter 8: How to Put Your Partner in a Sexual Trance

If you have been trying to discipline your sub but are still experiencing problems getting them into "Subspace" the trance state where they climax physically and emotionally (and not necessarily sexually) then it's time to review what most lacking Doms do wrong in the punishment phase.

First, understand that some experienced Doms claim that there are actually two stages of subspace - physiological and psychological.

Tip #34: Physiological subspace happens when there has been an abundance of pain play, usually from toys, not just the hand.

Make sure the punishment actually hurts and isn't too light. Keep the practice up for a significant period of time; usually ten minutes is all a sub needs to experience a new pain threshold, although this is not a hard rule.

Subs describe the feeling as a whole body buzzing, as well as a loss of focus on what is happening in their senses. It's almost as if the pain leaves them temporarily because of crossing a threshold.

Psychological subspace involves a strong attraction to a sub, one that is highly emotional and devotional. This may only be achievable after a history of building trust; though sometimes it can inexplicably happen after you just meet a person. This is also usually the state associated with **nonverbal or inarticulate behavior.**

Tip #35: Physiological subspace happens because of slowly but steadily crossing a pain threshold.

Psychological subspace happens on a very individual basis, and may involve different activities for different subs.

It may require one particularly erotic taboo being crossed, or maybe a long time of listening to their trusted Dom's voice. There is also such a thing as *Topspace*, which is the opposite trance—the ecstasy a Dom experiences when he reaches a psychologically induced trance state.

This strongly indicates a trance brought on by strong emotional and erotic exchanges, not necessarily just physical. The intensity level and intimacy between both participants reaches a spiritual level beyond the ordinary state of arousal.

What we do know about reaching this state is:

- The sub must want to experience it and not have any resistance

- There must be trust

- Endorphins and or adrenaline probably help bring the psychological subspace on; it may also involve other chemicals like serotonin and dopamine, present with feelings of love

- Some type of sensory deprivation may help, since this allows for a person's greater capacity to experienced altered states

- Stress and excitement releases endorphins

- The sub is adequately warmed up first; too much excitement or pain too soon is counteractive

- Sometimes the pre-foreplay and punishment stage can take hours; and coincidentally subspace can last for days

- It is usually associate with displays of affection

- The Dom must be very skilled and experienced in meeting the sub's needs completely

- An immersive environment (scents, music, sounds) and scene idea can help

Tip #36: Finding subspace is more a matter of responding to cues than finding a magical button.

Being attentive to the sub's behaviors, movements and sounds can be a good indicator that she is approaching subspace climax and you should keep steadily doing what you are doing—while also giving them a breather in between rounds of punishment.

Watch for the signs:

- The sub doesn't seem to think or speak clearly; they become slightly "high" or elusive in response.

- They clam up and want you, the Dom, to talk to them as a means of comfort

- They are more receptive to crude thoughts and vocabulary

- They revert back into more animalistic or primitive behaviors; grunting, growls and so on.

- They become more sensitive to light and movement

- The breathing of the sub becomes altered; usually her heart rate slows rather than speeding up from excitement. She breathes deeper and slower, requiring more oxygen.

- Their skin flushes and their eyes seem glazed

- Their voice changes; more throaty and moaning

It may well be a state of mind comparable to hypnosis, or detachment, out of body experience, and what is called "psychological compartmentalization." What is actually happening is that the sub is entering a state of mind where chemicals are taking over and she is experiencing a very mild hallucination state.

Identify these signs and keep going at a pace that is comfortable for the sub. That's all there is to it, though of course, a sub will "climax" in very different ways. And they're not necessarily orgasmic in nature. They may be rather quiet but internally explosive.

In our final chapter, we're going to discuss the more therapeutic motivations behind domination and how to better serve the sub with a mind towards cathartic self-improvement.

Chapter 9: How to Use BDSM Practices to Heal Someone's Pain

Before we explain the healing part of BDSM, let's start by saying BDSM is not a legitimate substitute for clinical therapy. BDSM is all about controlling irrational emotion while therapy is about logical solutions.

Healing basically means that the sub is trying to reconcile feelings and experiences of the past, typically in childhood, or maybe even fairly recent instances of relationship PTSD. They may confess what their bagging is, or you may have to figure it out.

Tip #37: BDSM healing usually involves letting go of guilty feelings regarding sex, or some other motivation.

This is fairly common among subs who were constantly disciplined via spankings or just guilted by verbal criticism. The goal of punishment is to allow her to face her mistakes, accept punishments and improve. Then, to be FORGIVEN for her past mistakes so she can MOVE ON.

Do you see the therapeutic value that punishment should have? It's not random. It serves a purpose in the sub's self-improvement.

You can make sorry excuses for punishing the sub, but they must always come with an explanation. This way, she is not confused about the reward-punishment system of discipline.

Tip #38: Anticipation for punishment is a great opportunity, and a little ritualistic planning goes a long way.

Making her wait for punishment, or having her choose her own implement of punishment, can help in creating embarrassment.

Tip #39: Lecturing the sub on why she is being punished is the parenting / teaching aspect of discipline, and deep down, is what the sub craves as the student. She wants to be taught how to improve and the lectures make this clear.

With punishment comes forgiveness, and then the love phase returns.

Tip #40: Focus her attention and give her small tasks to complete, increasing the difficulty steadily.

This involves a hypnotic trick of making her focus her attention on completing a task (say, balancing something on her head or shoulders without letting it fall) and then making it difficult for her to succeed because of your interfering actions. She is both trying to obey you, and follow your focus, while also anticipating punishment if she fails.

The scenario of forbidding the sub to make any sexual noises is another clever idea, since you can directly stimulate her while also punishing her if she fails to live up to your command. This sort of "Sweet Torture."

This does seem counteractive to being a good therapist or teacher, since you're tormenting your sub while also helping them work on their issues. But this is what makes BDSM practice unique. It's the only therapy that involves the naughty kind of "re-education" and mind control that other legitimate therapies forbid.

You're trespassing into forbidden psychology here; mind games, reprogramming, and slave-conditioning that the "real world" would never allow, except maybe in torturing prisoners of war.

The fact that you are role playing and all of this is voluntary allows you to get away with evil little tricks and mind games that you would never actually try with an innocent and non-consenting person. That's what makes it fun.

And sometimes the most radical forms of treatment are the best way to deal with a recurring mental issue. What could take a person a year in therapy to reconcile through conversation, could take only a month's worth of spanking and recreating past scenes in the sub's life that you are trying to deal with emotionally.

Helping the Sub with Long-Term Beneficial Discipline

The best Dom experience is going to be the one where you help the sub get over their personal problems and become a better person. This may seem strange to you, since this art is not considered a legitimate form of therapy or psychology. And it may even surprise Tops that are expecting to just find a slave to beat up on.

But yes, you can actually help subs with their personal problems and relationship baggage.

First consider the aims of legitimate therapy and then try to figure out how to apply them to the discipline and training of your sub.

Tip #41: Create a Dom curriculum based on what's going to help the sub (A) change, (B) cope or (C) feel better.

Ideally the teacher wants to help the student change for the better and eliminate nagging flaws "in real life" so that they can become happier and more productive. The same is true in BDSM lifestyle. You can teach the sub to change, whether it's eliminating bad personality traits (low self-esteem, immaturity, fear of intimacy) or changing their perspective.

If you can't change something you can at least help your sub learn how to cope with the stress or guilt of the past that still bothers her. This may actually involve teaching the sub more productive behaviors like exercising to relieve stress, exercising creativity, or simply speaking words of comfort to her during the aftercare.

You can also help the sub feel better by focusing on relieving or reducing anxiety that the sub feels about "real life", whether it's resulting from social isolation, anger, laziness, or difficulty in communicating her desires. The "punishments" and "rewards" you create can actually teach her life lessons and expose her to the things she really wants in her life, but fears achieving.

Cognitive therapy teaches that gradual exposure to phobias can work and help motivate patients to make slow but steady progress. They can actually get over their fears by confronting them in a controlled environment. You can do the same by gradually introducing your sub to the things she wants, but fears.

Tip #42: Do not punish the sub because of her fears or the failure to confront her fears.

Instead, reward her based on accomplishing landmarks that bring her closer to goal accomplishment. In contrast, punish her for the attitude that needs to change. She will gradually learn that seeking out rewards and taking on new challenges will be easier and more enjoyable than being punished for holding onto a destructive attitude.

Conclusion

We've reached the end of our book. Remember that finishing an advanced "billionaire" course in BDSM means that you are now ready to help someone realize their greatest potential. You are not merely interested in the sex—the sex is only the peripheral joy that can come from connecting with a sub and enjoying new layers of intimacy.

You also have the option of helping to transform the sub into becoming the better version of herself that she really wants to be. She may need help doing so. And she may even relapse in her life goals and come back to you.

Will you be there to help? It's a great privilege and honor to be of service to a sub. Your knowledge as a disciplinarian, a Master, a dominant, an Alpha and a teacher, will always be a commodity and a great value that subs will find very attractive.

This is going to be a life mission that brings you just as much joy as you give to others. Don't be intimidated by the thought of leadership. The world needs you and you know just what to do to help someone become their "personal best", don't you?

Other Books by Elizabeth Cramer

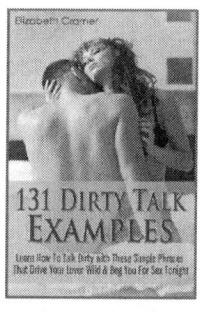

131 Dirty Talk Examples: Learn How To Talk Dirty with These Simple Phrases That Drive Your Lover Wild & Beg You For Sex Tonight

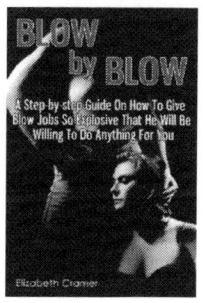

Blow By Blow - A Step-by-step Guide On How To Give Blow Jobs So Explosive That He Will Be Willing To Do Anything For You

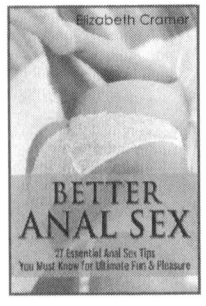 Better Anal Sex - 27 Essential Anal Sex Tips You Must Know for Ultimate Fun & Pleasure

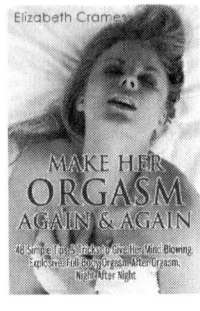 Make Her Orgasm Again and Again: 48 Simple Tips & Tricks to Give Her Mind-Blowing, Explosive, Full-Body Orgasm After Orgasm, Night After Night

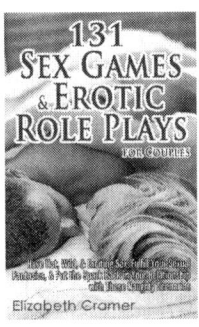 131 Sex Games & Erotic Role Plays for Couples: Have Hot, Wild, & Exciting Sex, Fulfill Your Sexual Fantasies, & Put the Spark Back in Your Relationship with These Naughty Scenarios

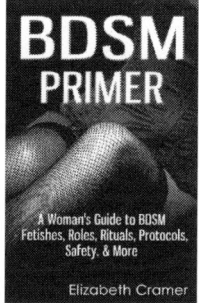

BDSM Primer - A Woman's Guide to BDSM - Fetishes, Roles, Rituals, Protocols, Safety, & More

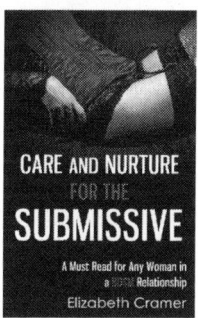

Care and Nurture for the Submissive - A Must Read for Any Woman in a BDSM Relationship

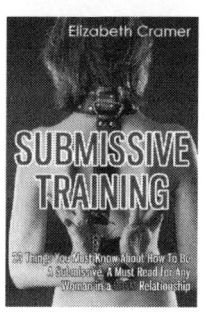

Submissive Training: 23 Things You Must Know About How To Be A Submissive. A Must Read For Any Woman In A BDSM Relationship

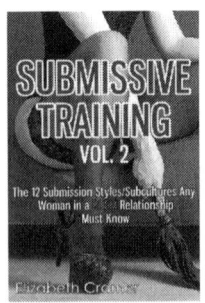
Submissive Training Vol. 2: The 12 Submission Styles/Subcultures Any Woman In A BDSM Relationship Must Know

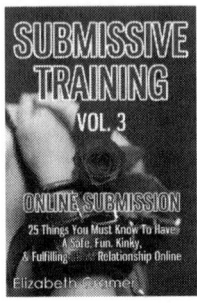
Submissive Training Vol. 3: Online Submission - 25 Things You Must Know To Have A Safe, Fun, Kinky, & Fulfilling BDSM Relationship Online

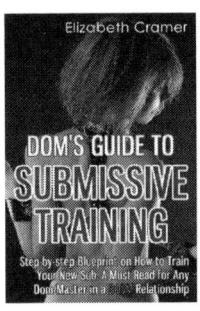
Dom's Guide To Submissive Training: Step-by-step Blueprint On How To Train Your New Sub. A Must Read For Any Dom/Master In A BDSM Relationship

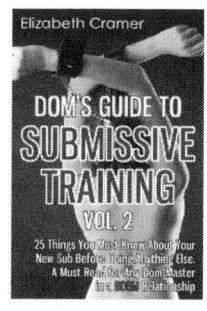
Dom's Guide To Submissive Training Vol. 2: 25 Things You Must Know About Your New Sub Before Doing Anything Else. A Must Read For Any Dom/Master In A BDSM Relationship

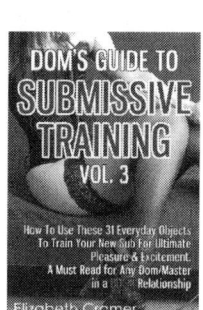
Dom's Guide To Submissive Training Vol. 3: How To Use These 31 Everyday Objects To Train Your New Sub For Ultimate Pleasure & Excitement. A Must Read For Any Dom/Master In A BDSM Relationship

Printed in Great Britain
by Amazon